International Baccala
Biology Option A
Neurobiology and Behaviour

Introduction

Welcome to the International Baccalaureate Revision Guide for Option A.

Sections A1 to A3 form the common core and sections A4 to A6 are the Additional Higher Level sections.

The format is the same as the Core Guides with key points, simple diagrams and large numbers of Grey Box Questions and Self-test quizzes.
Pale blue boxes contain information that helps with understanding by providing additional information. However you do not need to learn this.

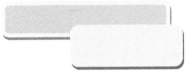

Other coloured boxes, such as these green and yellow ones, contain information that you do need to know.

The Option is tested, along with experimental skills and techniques linked to the Core material, in Paper 3.

I would greatly value any feedback on this revision guide. Please feel free to email me at Oxford Study Courses – osc@osc-ib.com

Ashby Merson-Davies

Contents

A1 Neural Development

Neurulation – Formation of the Neural Tube

In vertebrate animals after fertilisation the zygote divides by mitosis into a ball of cells called the blastula (blastocyst in mammals). The blastula then undergoes a process called gastrulation to form three layers of cells – ectoderm, mesoderm and endoderm. Each layer will differentiate into all the tissues and organs.

Annotate

neural plate

neural plate border

ectoderm

mesoderm

endoderm

A region of the ectoderm on the back differentiates to form the neural plate.

neural crest

neural groove

The neural plate folds inwards and the edges differentiate to form the neural crest.
Part of the mesoderm at the base of the neural groove begins to differentiate into the notochord.

The neural plate edges join to form a tube.
The two parts of the neural crest join and form a sheet between the ectoderm and neural tube.

neural tube

The neural tube becomes the spinal cord and brain.
The neural crest cells differentiate and develop into several cell types associated with the peripheral nervous system, e.g. myelin sheath cells, sensory, sympathetic and parasympathetic neurons – see page 8.
The somites formed from mesoderm develop into several tissues including the vertebrae, rib cage and skeletal muscle.
The notochord becomes part of the intervertebral disc.

somite

notochord

1.1 Development of the neural tube and associated tissues in the toad (*Xenopus*).

Neuron Development

❖ **Key points**

➢ Sensory, sympathetic and parasympathetic neurons develop from neural crest cells.
➢ Motor neurons develop within the spinal cord.
➢ An immature neuron consists of a cell body containing cytoplasm and a nucleus with a single short outgrowth called an axon.
➢ The axon grows in length and follows specific pathways to reach its target structure.
➢ These pathways are controlled by specific chemical markers.
➢ This target structure may be outside the neural tube.
➢ Some markers attract the growing tip of the neuron; other markers repel it.
➢ The axon carries information from the cell body and may develop many branches.
➢ Shorter, finer branches called dendrites grow out from the cell body and these carry information to the cell body.

Neuron Migration

❖ **Key points**

➢ Immature neurons can move from one region to another.
➢ This occurs frequently in the brain.
➢ Movement is brought about by the contraction/relaxation of actin fibres in the cytoplasm.
➢ Mature neurons do not normally move but damaged axons and dendrites can re-grow.

Synapse Development and Elimination

❖ **Key points**

➢ A developing neuron forms multiple synapses with other neurons or with effectors – see page 25.
➢ As the synapse forms, special structures are assembled, e.g. postsynaptic receptors and gated channels.
➢ Some neurons in the brain develop hundreds of synapses.
➢ This is called **neural networking** to allow complex transfer of information.
➢ Most synapses form during growth of the fetus but some can form in adulthood.
➢ When a synapse transfers an impulse a chemical marker is left which strengthens the synapse.
➢ Unused synapses do not accumulate these markers and eventually the synapse breaks down.

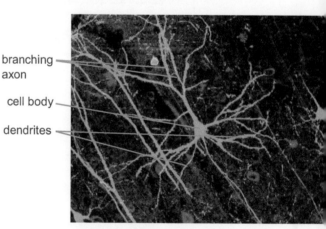

branching axon

cell body

dendrites

1.2 Image of a pyramidal neuron in the cerebral cortex of the mouse.

Neural Pruning

❖ **Key points**

➢ During fetal development of the brain more neurons form than are found in the adult brain.
➢ The unused neurons are lost either by programmed cell death (apoptosis) or neural pruning.
➢ Neural pruning involves loss of dendrites or axon branches as well as complete loss of the cell.

IB Option A © Ashby Merson-Davies

Plasticity of the Nervous System

❖ **Key points**

➢ Neural plasticity is the ability to modify the nervous system as a result of experiences.
➢ This can be done by:
   • Formation of new synapses and loss of others.
   • Neural apoptosis.
   • Neural pruning.
➢ In addition if a part of the brain has been damaged (e.g. by a stroke) adjacent neurons can take over the role of the lost neurons to restore some control.
➢ Recently stem cells have been found in some regions of the brain and these can reproduce and migrate to damaged areas to replace lost neurons.

Spina bifida

Look at the third diagram on page 3. The neural plate has folded over but not yet fused. In the fourth diagram it has and a tube has formed. Sometimes, usually in the lower back region, fusion does not occur and this prevents the vertebra, developing from the somites on each side, from enclosing it. The image on the left shows this. This very small gap is unlikely to produce any symptoms. However if the gap is larger then the spinal cord can protrude through it. This can produce severe disabilities.

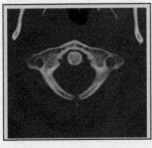

1.3 X-ray computed tomography scan of an unfused vertebral arch.

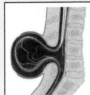

1.4 The spinal cord protrudes between the vertebrae.

Strokes

A stroke is loss of brain function due to a failure in blood supply resulting in oxygen starvation.
There are two types:
   • Ischemic – caused by a blockage, such as a blood clot.
   • Haemorrhagic – caused by a blood vessel bursting.
A very minor stroke may not be noticeable but larger ones can result in permanent loss of function of a part, or parts, of the body, or even death if a critical brain function is affected. In some cases other parts of the brain can take over the lost functions allowing the patient to regain some, or even all, of the functions. However this may involve relearning skills such as speech, writing, handling cutlery.

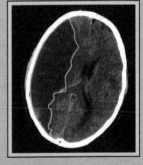

1.5 CT scan of an ischemic stroke. The dark area outlined in blue is the affected brain tissue.

1. Name the part of the ectoderm that develops into the neural tube.	2. Name the part of the ectoderm that develops into certain types of neuron.	3. Name the part of a neuron that carries information towards the cell body.
4. Name the part of a neuron that carries information away from the cell body.	5. State two structures that a neuron can form synapses with.	6. State two natural ways that neurons might be lost during development.

7. After a synapse has been formed what must happen in order for that synapse to be kept?	8. If the neural plate does not fuse together to form a tube the growing vertebra may not enclose it fully. What can this result in?

9. What is a stroke?	10. State two causes of a stroke.

Self-test quiz

1.   The neural plate develops into:
   a. The vertebrae.
   b. The notochord.
   c. The neural tube.
   d. Ectoderm.

2.   Which of the following statements about neuron development is true?
   a. The direction of growth of a neuron axon is determined by chemical stimuli.
   b. Electrical activity down a neuron stimulates its growth.
   c. Growth of axons from a neuron cell body follows random pathways.
   d. An axon forms a single synapse when it meets up with another neuron.

3.   Which of the following statements is not correct?
   a. Programmed cell death (apoptosis) is a way of removing neurons that are not used.
   b. Neurons develop multiple synapses but unused ones are removed.
   c. Immature neurons are able to move to different parts of the developing embryo.
   d. An axon forms numerous branches called dendrites to carry information to the cell body.

4.   Which of the following statements is not correct?
   a. Experiences are able to modify the nervous system by changing synaptic connections.
   b. Synapses can be strengthened by adding chemical markers.
   c. If a region of the brain is damaged, for example by a stroke, it cannot be repaired.
   d. Neural pruning leads to modifications in the synaptic connections in the brain.

5.   Spina bifida is a result of:
   a. The neural tube splitting into two regions.
   b. Failure of the neural tube to close over completely.
   c. Failure of the ectoderm to differentiate fully into the neural plate.
   d. Too many synaptic connections forming within the spinal cord.

A2 The Human Brain

❖ **Key points**

➢ The brain begins as an expansion of the anterior part the neural tube.
➢ There are three regions.

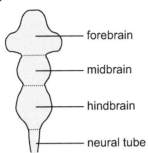

The developing brain viewed from above.

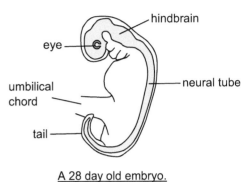

A 28 day old embryo.

➢ Different regions of the brain have specific functions.
➢ The cerebral cortex:
  • Forms a larger proportion of the brain.
  • Is more highly developed in humans compared to other animals.
  • Is enlarged principally by an increase in total area with extensive folding allowing it to fit within the cranium (skull).
➢ The cerebral hemispheres are responsible for higher order functions.
➢ The left cerebral hemisphere:
  • Receives sensory input:
    ▪ from the right side of the body
    ▪ from the right side of the visual field of <u>both</u> eyes (see page 17)
  • Controls muscle contraction in the right side of the body.
➢ The right cerebral hemisphere is the same but for the left side of the body.
➢ Brain metabolism requires large energy inputs.

> The cerebral cortex is the outer layer of the cerebral hemisphere. (Think of the cortex as a coat.)

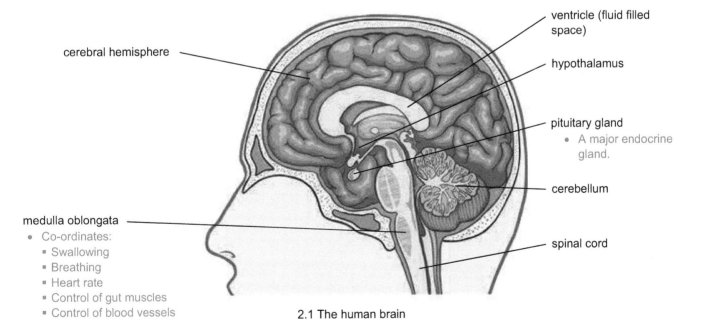

2.1 The human brain

medulla oblongata
• Co-ordinates:
  ▪ Swallowing
  ▪ Breathing
  ▪ Heart rate
  ▪ Control of gut muscles
  ▪ Control of blood vessels

> **The brain stem**
> The brain stem is made up of three regions connecting the spinal cord to the main part of the brain. The medulla, or medulla oblongata, is the one next to the spinal cord.

Organisation of the Nervous Systems

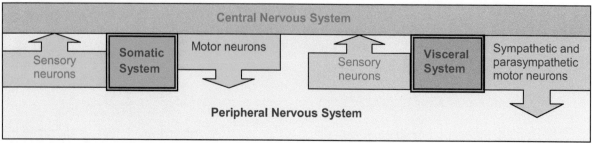

The somatic system is largely conscious and deals mainly with surface receptors and the skeletal muscles.

The visceral system is largely subconscious and deals with systems such as heart, gut, breathing. The motor neurons of the visceral system form the ANS. In general these are antagonistic, e.g. for the heart, sympathetic impulses speed it up and parasympathetic impulses slow it down. (*See core guide* SL *page 115,* HL *page 151.*)

The Autonomic Nervous System ANS

❖ **Key points**

➢ This controls the involuntary processes in the body – see medulla oblongata in the diagram on the previous page.
➢ The brain stem controls most of the ANS output.

Broca's area
- Part of the left cerebral hemisphere.
- Controls speech.
- Damage to this area results in the person knowing what they want to say but they can only make sounds and are unable to make meaningful words and sentences.

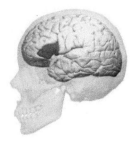

2.2 Broca's area

Nucleus accumbens ⬤ (in each hemisphere)
- These are the pleasure or reward centres of the brain.
- They release the neurotransmitter dopamine in response to various stimuli such as exercise, laughter, sex, and drugs including cocaine and heroine.

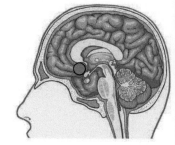

2.3 Nucleus accumbens

> You need to know the functions of three regions of the brain – **Broca's area, nucleus accumbens** and the **visual cortex**.

Primary Motor Cortex
Primary Somatosensory Cortex
Frontal Lobe
Parietal Lobe
Occipital Lobe
Olfactory Bulb
Cerebellum
Temporal Lobe
Spinal Cord

2.4 **The cerebral cortex**.
- This is divided into different lobes. (*You do not need to know the names.*)
- It is 2 – 4mm thick.
- During human evolution the thickness has not increased but the total surface area has.
- The cranium (skull) has enlarged to accommodate some of this but the enlargement has principally been by becoming highly folded.

- **The occipital lobe** is the **visual cortex** containing the visual processing centre which receives and processes information from the retinas of both eyes – see page 17.

- The olfactory bulb senses smell.
- The motor cortex deals with the planning, control, and execution of voluntary movements.
- The somatosensory cortex receives information from all the sensory receptors in the body, e.g. thermoreceptors, chemoreceptors, mechanoreceptors.

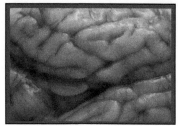

2.5 Close-up of the cerebral cortex showing the highly folded structure

IB Option A © Ashby Merson-Davies

Electroencephalography EEG

❖ Key Points

➤ This is looking at the electrical activity of the brain.
➤ Angelman syndrome is a neuro-genetic disorder with certain characteristics such as sleep disturbance, seizures, jerky movements (especially hand-flapping), and frequent laughter or smiling.
➤ It can be diagnosed from unusual patterns in an electroencephalogram.

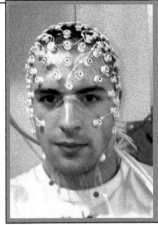

2.6 Sensors are set up over the skull to record an EEG.

The Pupil Reflex and Brain Death

❖ Key points

➤ The pupil reflex changes the diameter of the pupil to control the amount of light entering the eye.
➤ Constriction protects the retina from damage by excess light.
➤ Dilation allows sufficient light in for vision.
➤ Impulses from the retina are monitored for frequency by the brain stem.
➤ The brain stem is a part of the brain that includes the medulla. (See page 7).
➤ Monitoring is done regardless of whether the person is conscious or unconscious.
➤ A bright light is shone into the eye of the unconscious casualty.
➤ Failure of the pupil reflex in the casualty probably means brain death and the casualty is not likely to recover.
➤ This is because it indicates that if the brain stem is damaged the medulla is also probably damaged.
➤ The medulla oblongata regulates the basic life functions of breathing and heart rate.

Investigating Brain Function

❖ Key points of four procedures

Animal Experiments
➤ Usually involves surgery to remove part of the skull to access the brain.
➤ Animal must be alive.
➤ Different regions of the brain are stimulated and the response of the animal observed.
➤ Primates were often used which raised ethical issues given their genetic similarity to humans and the pain and suffering caused.
➤ Example: Pierre Flourens in the 1820s showed that removing thin slices of tissue from the cerebellum of rabbits and birds resulted in the animals displaying a lack of muscular co-ordination and poor balance but no other obvious effects.

Lesions

 - ➢ A lesion is a damaged part of the brain.
 - ➢ This may be due to a stroke, tumour, accident or deliberate injury.
 - ➢ The change in ability of the person or experimental animal before and after lesion formation can be used to deduce the function of that region.
 - ➢ The lesion may be produced by drilling a hole in the skull of the anaesthetised animal, inserting an electrode into a specific part of the brain and using an electric impulse to destroy the tissue around the electrode tip.
 - ➢ Example: in rats a lesion in a specific part of the hypothalamus causes over-eating whereas a lesion in a different part caused the rats, initially, to refuse all food.
 - ➢ Lesions in humans have been done for therapeutic purposes – certain nerve fibres linking opposite sides of the brain have been cut in an attempt to reduce epileptic seizures.

Autopsy

 - ➢ This is examination of a body after death.
 - ➢ The position of a lesion in the brain can be related to any unusual behavioural traits shown by the person when they were alive.
 - ➢ Behavioural changes can also be associated with changes to the chemical make-up of the brain and also physical changes.
 - ➢ Example: variant CJD is caused by the formation of prion proteins in the brain. Microscopic holes are characteristic in prion-affected tissue sections, causing the tissue to develop a spongy appearance. (Variant CJD is the human form of BSE).

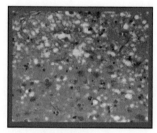

2.7 A micrograph of brain tissue of a BSE-affected cow showing the microscopic holes.

Functional Magnetic Resonance Imaging (fMRI)

 - ➢ The fMRI scanner detects differences in oxygenated and deoxygenated blood.
 - ➢ It can detect active brain tissue of only a few square mm.
 - ➢ Brain tissue becomes active when stimulated and oxygen consumption increases.
 - ➢ This causes an increase in blood flow.
 - ➢ Change in oxygen consumption in the active neural area occurs 1 - 5 seconds after the stimulus.
 - ➢ Example shown on the right.

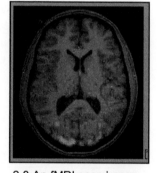

2.8 An fMRI scan image.

While lying in the FMRI scanner the subject watched a screen which alternated between showing a visual stimulus and being dark every 30 seconds. Note the increased blood flow (red and yellow) in the visual cortex (see pages 8 and 17).

Correlation between brain size and body size

 - ❖ Key points

 - ➢ The relationship between brain size and body size shows a positive correlation.

Species	Brain : body ratio (E:S)
small birds	1 : 14
mouse	1 : 40
human	1 : 40
cat	1 : 110
dog	1 : 125
lion	1 : 550
elephant	1 : 560
horse	1 : 600
shark	1 : 2500

The table shows the approximate simple ratios of brain mass to body mass.

IB Option A © Ashby Merson-Davies

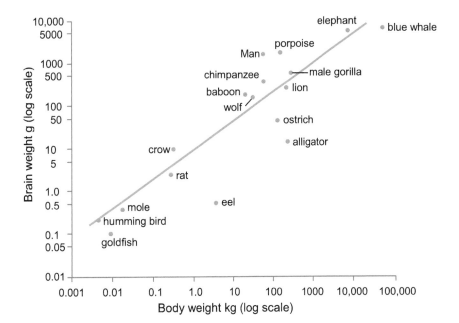

Graph of the simple E:S ratio using a log scale. This clearly shows the positive correlation.

➤ The simple E:S ratio can be misleading as it gives no indication of cognitive ability.
➤ The table shows mouse and human have the same E:S ratio and small birds have a relatively larger brain mass compared to humans. (Birds have hollow bones, some of which have air sacks in them, which makes them much lighter relative to other animals of the same size).
➤ The brain consists of interconnecting neurons that store and process information along with supporting cells.
➤ There can be a large increase in the number of neurons with only a small increase in brain size.
➤ A better value for comparing animals is the encephalisation quotient, EQ.
➤ The mean EQ for mammals is 1.

Species	EQ
Man	>7
Dolphin	4.6
Chimpanzee	2.4
Elephant	2.0
Dog	1.2
Cat	1.0
Horse	0.9
Mouse	0.5

• This table relates much better to perceived intelligence.
• Man is a long way in front, and dolphins are well known for their intelligence.
• Social animals have a higher EQ to allow them to interact within a group.
• Carnivores have a higher EQ associated with hunting skills.
• Herbivores have a lower EQ.

Brain function

❖ **Key points**

➤ Although particular regions of the brain can be assigned specific functions, brain imagery shows that some activities are spread over other parts of the brain.
➤ Following damage to the brain, such as with a stroke, other parts of the brain can be reorganised to take over the functions from the damaged parts.

1. Label on the dotted lines.

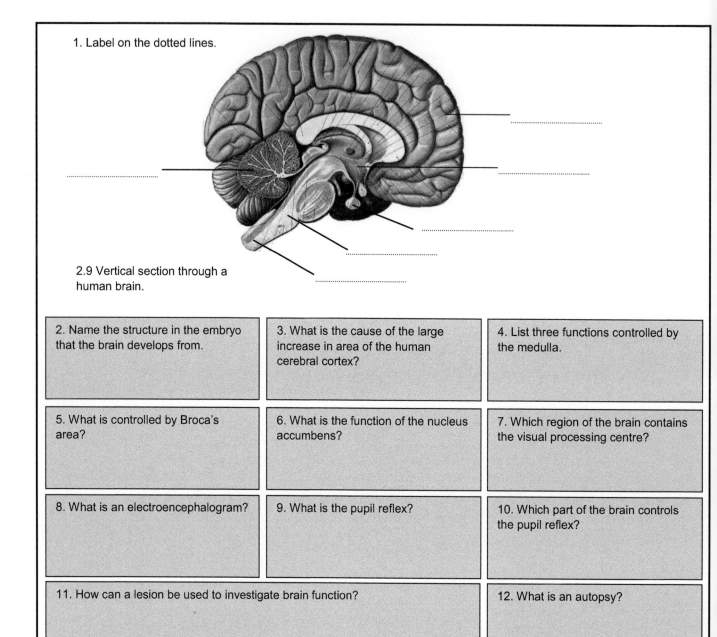

2.9 Vertical section through a human brain.

2. Name the structure in the embryo that the brain develops from.	3. What is the cause of the large increase in area of the human cerebral cortex?	4. List three functions controlled by the medulla.
5. What is controlled by Broca's area?	6. What is the function of the nucleus accumbens?	7. Which region of the brain contains the visual processing centre?
8. What is an electroencephalogram?	9. What is the pupil reflex?	10. Which part of the brain controls the pupil reflex?

11. How can a lesion be used to investigate brain function?	12. What is an autopsy?

13. How can an fMRI scan be used to investigate brain function?	14. State one other way brain function has been investigated.

15. What type of correlation is shown by a graph of brain size v body size?

IB Option A © Ashby Merson-Davies

Self-test quiz

1. Which line in the table is correct?

		Brain stem	Left cerebral hemisphere	Right cerebral hemisphere
a.		Controls autonomic functions	Receives sensory input from the left side of the body.	Receives sensory input from the right side of the body.
b.		Controls breathing and heart rate.	Receives sensory input from the right side of the body.	Receives sensory input from the left side of the body.
c.		Controls autonomic functions.	Receives sensory input from both sides of the body.	Receives sensory input from both sides of the body.
d.		Controls speech functions.	Receives input from the right side of the visual field of both eyes.	Receives input from the left side of the visual field of both eyes.

2. The cerebral cortex is:
    a. The outer layer of the cerebral hemispheres.
    b. The outer layer of the cerebellum.
    c. The region where the spinal cord enters the skull.
    d. The region of the brain just above the pituitary gland.

3. Which part of the brain is responsible for higher order functions?
    a. Cerebellum.
    b. Broca's area.
    c. Nucleus accumbens.
    d. Cerebral hemispheres.

4. Which of the following statements about the autonomic nervous system (ANS) is correct?
    a. It has sensory and motor neurons associated with sensory receptors in the skin.
    b. It is composed of motor neurons that control subconscious functions of the body.
    c. Sensory neurons of the ANS monitor heart rate.
    d. Sympathetic sensory neurons connect with parasympathetic motor neurons in the brain stem.

5. Which part of the brain is the reward / pleasure centre?
    a. Nucleus accumbens.
    b. Broca's area.
    c. Medulla oblongata.
    d. Cerebellum.

6. Which region of the brain contains the visual cortex?
    a. Cerebral cortex.
    b. Occipital lobe.
    c. Cerebral hemispheres.
    d. Brain stem.

7. Which of the following statements about the pupil reflex is correct?
    a. It only occurs when a person moves from a dark room to a brightly lit room.
    b. It is a decrease in the diameter of the lens to reduce the amount of light entering the eye.
    c. It occurs when a person is unconscious as well as when conscious.
    d. It only occurs in a conscious person.

8. The pupil reflex is controlled by:
    a. The brain stem.
    b. The cerebral cortex.
    c. The cerebellum.
    d. The nucleus accumbens.

9. Lesions can be used to help determine brain function because:
    a. They can be easily removed by surgery.
    b. They only occur in specific regions of the brain.
    c. They always have the same effect on the functioning of the brain.
    d. They are damaged parts of the brain and can be correlated with a change in the way the animal / human behaves.

10. Which of the following statements about functional magnetic resonance imaging (fMRI) is correct?
    a. It measures an increase in the electrical activity of a stimulated area of the brain.
    b. It measures an increase in the flow of oxygenated blood to an active area of the brain.
    c. It measures a decrease in the flow of oxygenated blood to an active area of the brain.
    d. It measures a change in the carbon dioxide content of the blood in an active region of the brain.

A3 Perception of Stimuli

Receptors

❖ **Key points**

➢ These detect changes in the environment.
➢ The environment can be external or internal.

	Mechanoreceptors	**Chemoreceptors**	**Thermoreceptors**	**Photoreceptors**
Stimulus	Mechanical movement; pressure; forces	Chemicals	Temperature	Light
Types	Stretch receptors in muscles are used to position muscles in co-ordinated movements.	Taste and smell receptors on the tongue and in the nose (olfactory receptors). The stomach wall has receptors that can detect amino acids. Carbon dioxide receptors in carotid bodies on carotid arteries lead to regulation of breathing.	Hypothalamus measures temperature of blood for temperature homeostasis. The skin contains hot and cold receptors.	Rods and cones in the retina.

The Human Eye

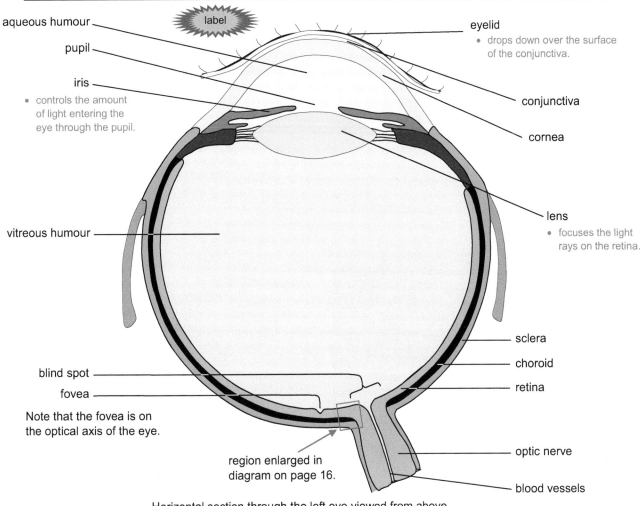

Horizontal section through the left eye viewed from above.

Rods and Cones

	Rods	**Cones**
Sensitivity	High: used in dim light.	Low: used in bright light.
Types	One type detects all wavelengths but in monochrome.	Three types absorbing maximally at blue, green and red regions of the spectrum.
Distribution	Not present in the fovea.*	Not present at the very edge of the retina.

* If you look directly at a dim star you cannot see it because the image falls on the fovea where there are only the less sensitive cones. Look just to the side of it so the image falls outside the fovea and you can now see it.

Hint – rod = dim : cones = colour

The retina

- Rod cells are connected in large groups to a single bipolar neuron (only 3 shown here).
- Far fewer cone cells are connected to one ganglion cell.

This makes colour vision sharper. In low light when only the rods are working objects are more blurred. In the fovea as few as 5 cone cells are connected to one ganglion cell.

- The blind spot is where ganglion cells pass into the optic nerve through the layer of rod and cone cells.

The part of the image falling in this region is not detected. However the blind spot is in a different position in each eye (see page 15) so a different part of the image falls on each blind spot. Thus the left eye 'fills in' for the right eye and vice versa.

- Direction of light entering eye.

Any light not absorbed by the rod or cone cells is absorbed by the black pigment of the choroid layer.

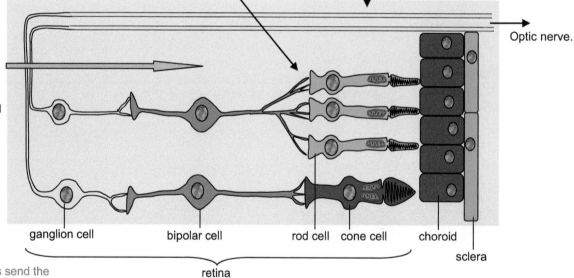

Optic nerve.

ganglion cell   bipolar cell   rod cell   cone cell   choroid

sclera

retina

- Ganglion cells send the impulses from the ganglion cells to the brain via the optic nerve
- Bipolar cells send the impulses from the rods and cones to the ganglion cells

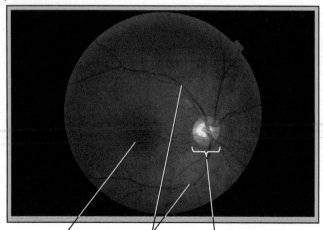

fovea   blood vessels   blind spot

3.1 Human retina photographed through the iris.

Find your blind spot
Hold the book in front of you about 50cm away. Close your left eye and look at the cross with your right eye. Slowly bring the book towards you. At around 35 – 40cm the blue spot will disappear. Try swinging your head from side to side but keep looking at the cross – you still won't be able to see the spot. Try it the other way round as well.

Notice that the blood vessels pass through the centre of the blind spot and the neurons form a white ring around them – see page 15.

IB Option A © Ashby Merson-Davies

Optic Nerves and the Visual Cortex

➢ Information from the right visual field from both eyes is sent to left part of the visual cortex and vice versa.
➢ Note how the optic nerves join together and cross over in the optic chiasma.

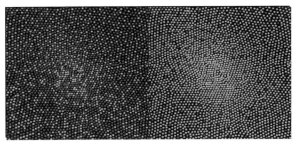

Colour vision

➢ There are three different cone types with peak sensitivity in the red, green and blue parts of the spectrum.
➢ All other colours are made from blending these three.
➢ This is called **trichromatic vision**.
➢ Red-green colour blindness is caused by a genetic fault in one or more genes associated with the red or green cones.
➢ The degree of loss of sensitivity to red or green colours is variable depending on the genetic fault.
➢ The fault could be:
   • Abnormal photopigment in the red cones or in the green cones.
   • No red cones or no green cones.

3.2 This is an illustration of the distribution of cone cells in the fovea of an individual with normal colour vision (left), and a person who has a form of red-green colour blindness called protanopia – they have no red cones.

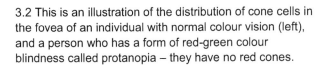

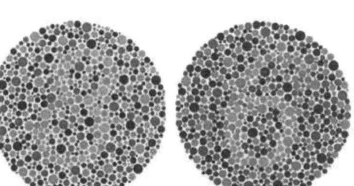

3.3 These are four plates from the Ishihara test. The table shows the number that would be seen by a person with normal colour vision and a person who is red-green colour blind.

	Normal colour vision	Red-green colour blind
Top left	8	3
Top right	6	5
Bottom left	5	2
Bottom right	15	17

Important: Due to limitations in colour printing these reproduced plates should NOT be used as an actual test of colour vision.

Red-green colour blindness is caused by a recessive gene mutation on the X chromosome. Thus it is more common in males than females – *see* Core Guide, SL *page 182*, HL *page 259*.

Olfactory Receptors

❖ **Key points**

➢ These are chemoreceptors found in the epithelium of the nose.
➢ Humans have about 100 - 200 that can detect an estimated 10,000 different odours.
➢ The cilia of the olfactory cell contain the odorant receptor proteins.
➢ Each protein is coded for by a different gene.
➢ Each olfactory cell only expresses one type of protein.

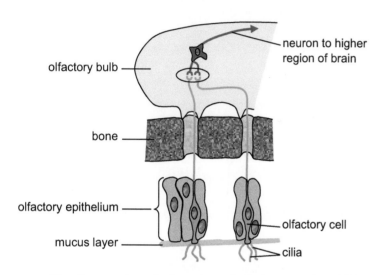

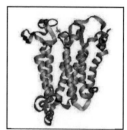

3.4 The structure of an odorant receptor protein.

Humans have about 500-750 odorant genes but only express about 100-200. Compared to other mammals our sense of smell is poor.
The structure of the proteins is closely related to the structure of the photoreceptor protein rhodopsin.

The diagram shows just one type of olfactory receptor which will be specific for a particular chemical odour or odorant. These will be distributed in groups in the nasal mucosa but are all connected to a single neuron to the brain.

| 1. Sensory receptors | Complete the shaded boxes using one example for each. | | | |

	Mechanoreceptors			
Stimulus	mechanical deformation	chemicals	temperature	light
Types				

2. Which type of light receptor is found in the fovea?	3. Which type of light receptor is receptive at low light intensities?	4. Which type of light receptor responds to colour?
5. Information from which part of the visual field is received by the left visual cortex?	6. How many types of colour receptor are there?	7. What causes red-green colour blindness?

IB Option A © Ashby Merson-Davies

8. The Eye

Label the drawing of the eye in the 15 places indicated.

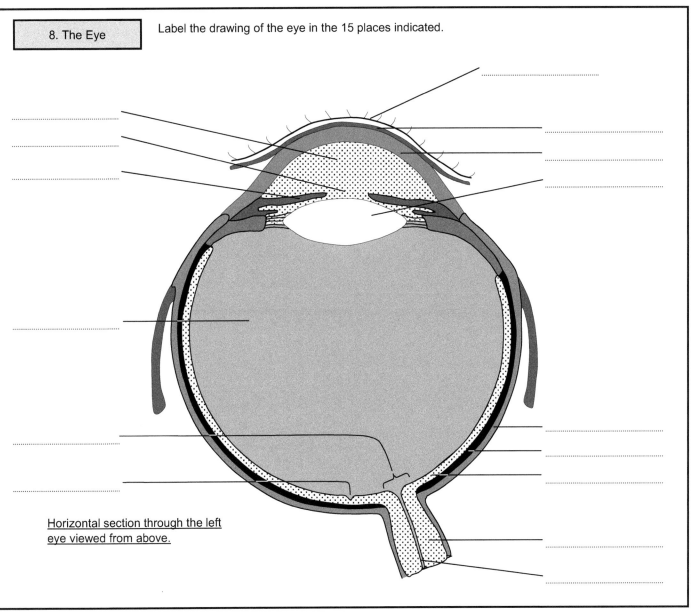

Horizontal section through the left
eye viewed from above.

9. The Eye

Add relevant annotations in the three boxes and add labels on the 6 dotted lines.

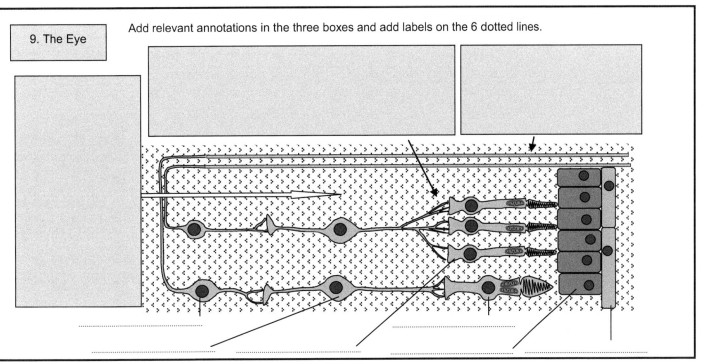

The Human Ear

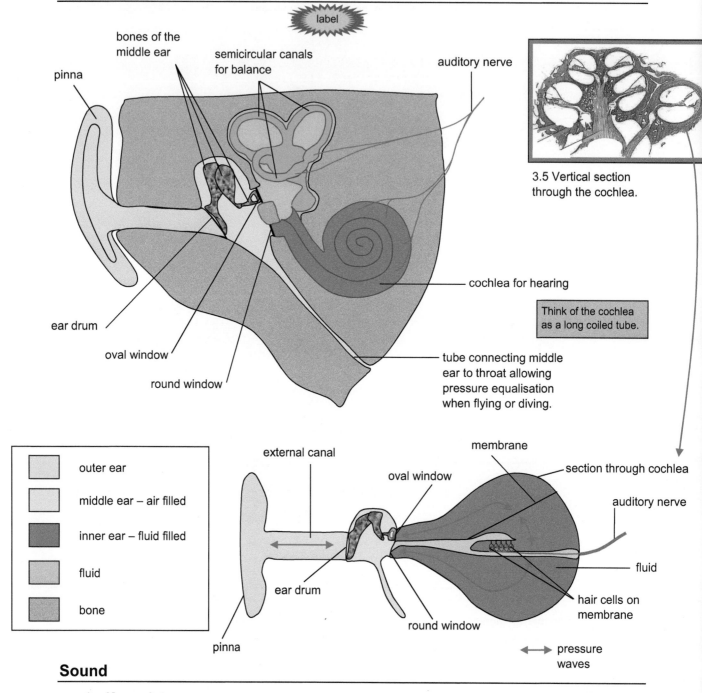

label

bones of the middle ear

semicircular canals for balance

auditory nerve

pinna

ear drum

oval window

round window

cochlea for hearing

tube connecting middle ear to throat allowing pressure equalisation when flying or diving.

3.5 Vertical section through the cochlea.

Think of the cochlea as a long coiled tube.

outer ear

middle ear – air filled

inner ear – fluid filled

fluid

bone

external canal

oval window

membrane

section through cochlea

auditory nerve

fluid

hair cells on membrane

ear drum

pinna

round window

pressure waves

Sound

❖ **Key points**

➢ The pinna collects the sounds from the environment.
➢ These sounds are in the form of pressure waves.
➢ An air pressure wave passes down the external canal.
➢ This pushes on the **ear drum** which moves the **bones in the middle ear**.
➢ These bones have several functions:
  • The first bone is attached to the ear drum and the third to the oval window
  • They act as levers which increases the force transmitted from the ear drum to the oval window.
  • Muscles attaching them to the skull can contract as a result of a very loud sound and this prevents excessive movement of the oval window.

Animals which are hunted, such as deer, rabbits or hares, have large and mobile pinnae which they use to detect sounds from predators.

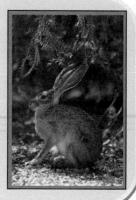

3.6 A hare (*Lepus* sp).

IB Option A © Ashby Merson-Davies

➤ The bones push on the **oval window** which causes a pressure wave in the fluid-filled **cochlea**.
➤ The **round window** moves in sympathy with the oval window, i.e. as the oval window moves in the round window moves out and vice versa.
➤ This allows the fluid in the cochlea to move freely backwards and forwards.
➤ This fluid movement pushes on the membrane on which the **hair cells** sit.
➤ These hair cells are a type of **mechanoreceptor**; (*see page 15*).
➤ Movement of the hairs triggers nerve impulses in the **auditory nerve**.
➤ The auditory nerve transmits the impulses to the **auditory cortex.**
➤ The pitch of a sound is determined by its frequency. Different frequencies travel different distances along the cochlea – the lower the frequency the further it travels.
➤ The louder the sound the greater the amplitude of the pressure wave and the greater the frequency of impulses sent to the brain.

Movement of the Head

❖ **Key points**

➤ The three fluid-filled semicircular canals are on three different axes or planes.
➤ They contain hair cells.
➤ When the head moves the fluid in one or more canals moves and stimulates the hair cells.
➤ This information is transmitted via the auditory nerve to the brain.

> If you spin round and round and then stop you feel dizzy and cannot walk straight. This is because the fluid in the horizontal semicircular canal continues to move which tells the brain you are still spinning.

Cochlear Implant

❖ **Key points**

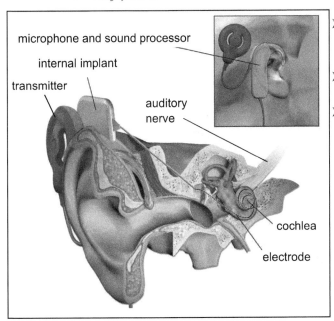

3.7 A cochlear implant.

➤ In some cases of deafness a simple hearing aid placed in the auditory canal can amplify sounds so they can be heard.
➤ In other cases the hair cells in the cochlea are not functioning and a hearing aid will not help.
➤ A cochlear implant is a surgically implanted electronic device that connects directly to the auditory nerve.
  • The microphone picks up the sounds.
  • The sound processor selects speech frequencies and filters out non speech frequencies.
  • The speech frequencies are sent to the transmitter.
  • The internal implant then sends the speech frequencies to the auditory nerve.
➤ An implant is especially important if a child is born deaf as it will allow them to develop listening and speech skills and therefore attend a normal school.

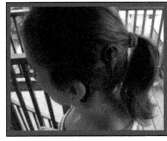

3.8 A young girl with a cochlear implant.

10. The Ear   Label the drawing in the 9 places indicated.

11. The Ear   Label the drawing in the 9 places indicated.

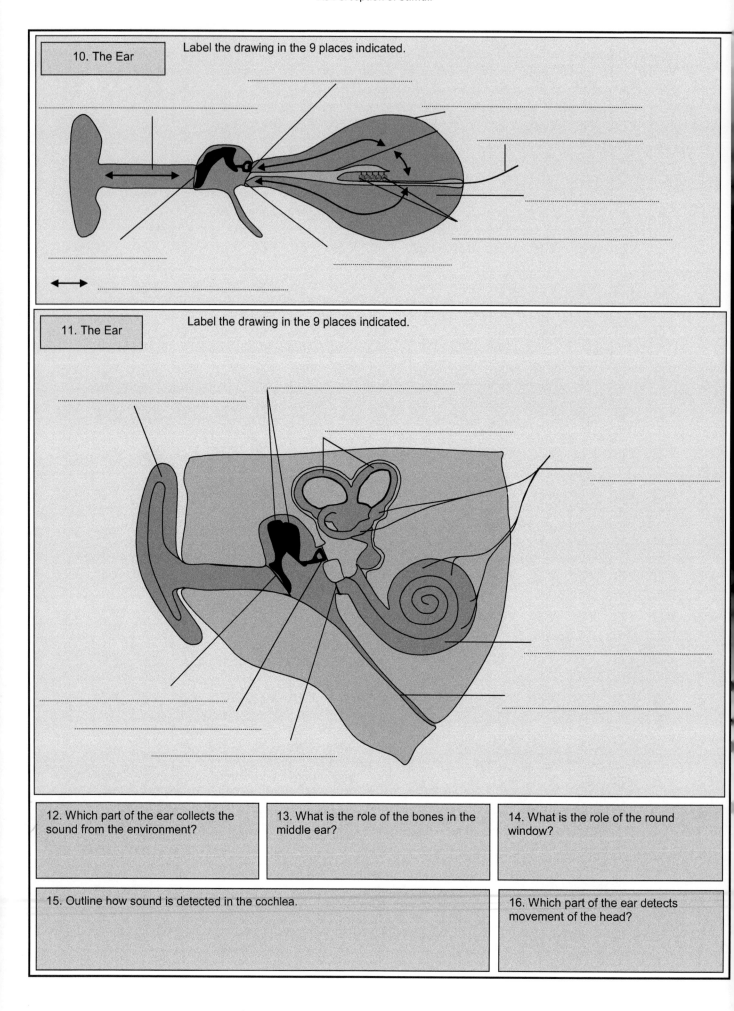

12. Which part of the ear collects the sound from the environment?

13. What is the role of the bones in the middle ear?

14. What is the role of the round window?

15. Outline how sound is detected in the cochlea.

16. Which part of the ear detects movement of the head?

Self-test quiz

1. Which of the following is a mechanoreceptor?
   a. Carbon dioxide receptor in the carotid artery.
   b. Stretch receptor in muscle.
   c. Cone cell in the retina.
   d. Olfactory receptor in the nose.

2. Which of the following descriptions of the structure of the eye is correct?
   a. As light enters the eye it passes through the cornea, then the conjunctiva, then the lens.
   b. The outer layer is the sclera and the inner layer is the retina.
   c. The vitreous humour is in front of the lens and the aqueous humour is behind the lens.
   d. The iris is the hole in the centre of the pupil through which light enters the eye.

3. Which of the following statements is correct?
   a. The most sensitive region of the retina is the fovea because it contains both rods and cones.
   b. The blind spot is a ring around the fovea where there are no photoreceptor cells.
   c. The most sensitive region of the retina is the fovea because it contains only cones.
   d. The blind spot is the area on the fovea which contains only rods.

4. Which is the correct sequence of retinal cells through which light passes to reach the choroid layer?
   a. Ganglion cells; bipolar cells; photoreceptor cells; choroid.
   b. Photoreceptor cells; bipolar cells; ganglion cells; choroid.
   c. Bipolar cells; ganglion cells; photoreceptor cells; choroid.
   d. Photoreceptor cells; ganglion cells; bipolar cells; choroid.

5. Which of the following statements is correct?
   a. The left visual cortex receives information from the left visual field of both eyes and vice versa.
   b. The right visual cortex receives information from the left eye and vice versa.
   c. The right visual cortex receives information from the right eye and vice versa.
   d. The left visual cortex receives information from the right visual field of both eyes and vice versa.

6. Which of the following statements is correct?
   a. Colour vision is due to three different types of rod photoreceptor cells.
   b. Colour photoreceptor cells are only found in the fovea.
   c. Colour vision is due to three different types of cone photoreceptor cells.
   d. Colour vision is brought about by interaction between rod and cone cells.

7. Which of the following about the pathway of sound / pressure waves entering the ear is correct?
   a. Pinna – oval window – round window – ear drum – bones of the middle ear.
   b. Pinna – ear drum – bones of the middle ear – oval window – round window.
   c. Pinna – ear drum – bones of the middle ear – round window – oval window.
   d. Pinna – round window – bones of the middle ear – oval window – ear drum.

8. Which of the following statements about sound perception is correct?
   a. When the pinna is moved by sound pressure waves it causes the bones of the middle ear to move.
   b. Movement of the hair cells in the cochlea stimulates nerve impulses in the auditory nerve.
   c. When the bones of the middle ear move the oval window inwards the round window moves inwards,
   d. The hair cells on the membrane in the inner ear are chemoreceptors.

9. Which of the following statements is correct?
   a. The semicircular canals contain mechanoreceptor cells.
   b. Movement of the head is detected by sensory cells in the cochlea.
   c. Movement of the oval window moves the fluid in the semicircular canals causing nerve impulses to be sent along the auditory nerve.
   d. The auditory nerve is connected to both oval and round windows and detects movement of these.

10. Which of the following statements about the bones of the middle ear is correct?
    a. Movement of the muscles attached to them allow the movement of the ear drum to be transferred to the oval window.
    b. Movement of the muscles attached to them allow the movement of the ear drum to be transferred to the round window.
    c. They act as levers to transmit and amplify the movement between the ear drum and the oval window.
    d. They act as levers to transmit and amplify the movement between the oval window and the round window.

11. A cochlear implant is:
    a. An electronic device to help someone who is unable to balance properly.
    b. A special type of hearing aid for a person whose cochlear hair cells are not functioning correctly.
    c. A special type of hearing aid for a person whose auditory nerve has become detached from the cochlear.
    d. A special type of hearing aid for a person whose auditory nerve has been damaged.

HL only
A4 Innate and Learned Behaviour

Innate Behaviour
➢ Is inherited from parents.
➢ Therefore develops independently from the environment.
➢ Occurs in all members of a species despite natural variation in environmental influences.
➢ Is in the form of reflexes.

Reflexes

❖ **Key points**

➢ These are involuntary responses.
➢ They are controlled by the autonomic nervous system.

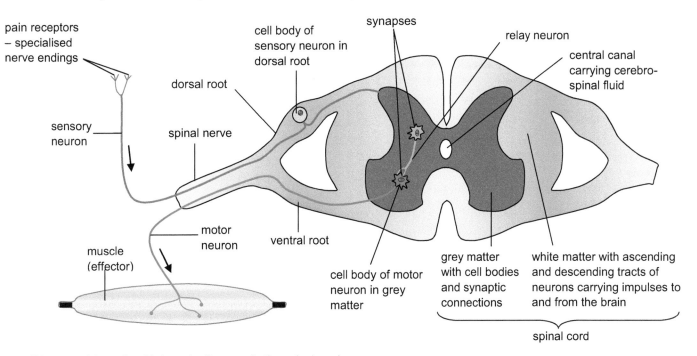

Diagram of the pain withdrawal reflex arc via the spinal cord.

❖ **Key components**

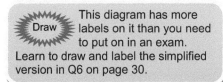
This diagram has more labels on it than you need to put on in an exam. Learn to draw and label the simplified version in Q6 on page 30.

➢ **Receptor**
• Specialised cell or nerve ending.
• Detects a specific stimulus.
• Detects internal and external stimuli.
➢ **Sensory neuron**
• Carries nerve impulses from the receptor to the central nervous system.
➢ **Relay neuron**
• Carries nerve impulses from the sensory to the motor neuron.
• Links up with other relay neurons to carry information up and down the spinal cord, e.g. to the memory centres of the brain.
➢ **Motor neuron**
• Carries nerve impulses from the central nervous system to the effector.
➢ **Synapses**
• Connect neurons together.
• Control how the information is passed from one neuron to the next.
• Uses chemicals called neurotransmitters.
➢ **Effector**
• Muscle or secretory gland.
• Carries out a response to the stimulus.

Learned Behaviour
> - Is the acquisition of skill or knowledge.
> - It depends on memory, which is the process of encoding, storing and then accessing the relevant information.
> - It develops as a result of experience.
> - These experiences may come:
>   - From the physical environment.
>   - From observing another individual.
> - Four types are:
>   - Reflex conditioning.
>   - Operant conditioning.
>   - Imprinting.
>   - Latent learning.

Reflex Conditioning

Reflex Conditioning:
The modification of behaviour in an animal in response to a repeated stimulus in such a way that the stimulus and response become associated.

❖ **Key points**

> - Also called Pavlovian conditioning after the Russian psychologist Pavlov who investigated saliva flow in dogs.
> - He presented meat powder, the unconditioned stimulus, to the dog.
> - The dog responded by increased saliva flow, the unconditioned response.
> - He then rang a bell, at the same time as presenting the meat powder.
> - After several repeats the bell alone, the conditioned stimulus, would cause the dog to increase saliva flow, the conditioned response.

Operant Conditioning

Operant Conditioning:
A learning mechanism in which the reward follows only after the correct behavioural response.

❖ **Key points**

> - Investigations by the American psychologist Skinner.
> - He placed a rat in a special box (now called a Skinner box).
> - As the rat explored the box it would at first accidentally press a lever.
> - Pressing the lever released a pellet of food.
> - Initially the rat would ignore the lever, simply eat the food and continue moving.
> - Soon the rat learnt to associate pressing the lever with the appearance of the food.
> - Pressing the lever is called the operant response.
> - The appearance of food is called the reinforcement.

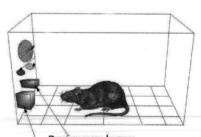

Response lever

Food dispenser

4.1 A Skinner box.

Imprinting

❖ **Key points**

> **Imprinting:**
> An attachment to an object encountered during a sensitive time period, often immediately after birth.

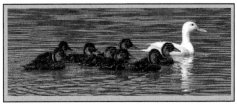

> ➤ Investigations by the German ethologist Konrad Lorenz. It makes sense for an offspring to be able to recognise a parent that will supply it with food and protection.
> ➤ During the sensitive time period the animal responds to the sign stimulus which is the nearest moving object.
> ➤ The sign stimulus triggers the innate releasing mechanism that results in the particular species specific behaviour.

4.2 Ducklings imprinted on their surrogate mother.

> ➤ As an animal matures it grows out of this initial species specific behaviour, but modifies it to form attachments to other individuals and develop preferences.
> ➤ Lorenz hatched some geese in an incubator and so he was the sign stimulus.
> ➤ Newly hatched geese follow their mother, so in this case the species specific behaviour was to follow Lorenz.
> ➤ As adults though they were unable to develop normal relationships with other geese.
> ➤ Hence the initial sign stimulus may have an important role in adult life.

Latent Learning - Development of Birdsong

❖ **Key points**

> **Latent Learning:**
> Learning which is not apparent in the learner's behaviour at the time of learning, but which develops later when a suitable motivation occurs.

> ➤ Adult songbirds have a species-specific song used in territorial display and courtship.
> ➤ In some species it is entirely innate but in others there is a part which is learned.
> ➤ Example: White-crowned sparrow, *Zonotrichia leucophrys*.
>   • In nature the nestlings will hear the songs of mature males.
>   • A young bird leaves the nest but does not become sexually mature until the following spring.
>   • A male that has been hatched and reared in isolation can sing but not the species-specific song.
>   • Some components of what it sings are species-specific, indicating they are innate, but they are not the right length or in the right order.
>   • If a young bird hears the adult species-specific song it can then repeat that song the following spring. If a young bird hears the adult song but its hearing is blocked before spring it is unable to repeat the song.
>   • This means it has to hear its own singing and match what it hears with what was programmed into its memory as a young bird.
>   • If a young bird hears the adult song but its hearing is blocked <u>after</u> it has started to sing in the spring it is able to continue to repeat the song correctly even though it can no longer hear itself.
>   • Thus there are two learning phases in this bird:
>   ▪ The first when it is young.
>   ▪ The second at the start of sexual maturity.

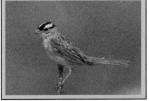

4.3a White-crowned sparrow, (*Zonotrichia leucophrys*).

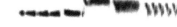
A sonogram of the tutor.

Early sonogram of the pupil.

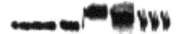
Final sonogram of the pupil.

4.3b These three sonograms show the two stages of song learning in a young white crowned sparrow.

Other examples of learning

Learning and Survival

❖ **Points for discussion**

➢ A greater range of behaviours can be acquired over time than could be acquired by natural selection.

➢ More complex behaviour can be developed over time which can confer great survival value for the species.

➢ Communication means information can be passed on to later generations.

➢ Learning reduces the amount of non-adaptive behaviour, e.g. not running away from predators, which increases the chances of survival.

➢ In higher organisms, e.g. primates, where there are many complex behaviours, it is very inefficient for each behaviour to be controlled by genes. It is much better to have a few genes which give the ability to learn.

➢ It allows behaviour to be tailored to a particular environment, e.g. a predator could switch to different forms of prey if its main source became scarce.

Examples:

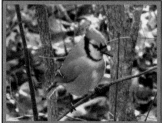

4.4 Blue jay.

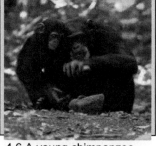

4.6 A young chimpanzee watching its mother use a rock to break open a seed.

▪ An inexperienced caged Blue Jay will take a Milkweed butterfly if offered but spit it out due to its horrible taste. If offered another one it will refuse.

▪ Alaskan Brown bears head towards particular rivers at the same time as salmon are moving up the rivers to spawn. The cubs learn this from their mothers.

4.5 Brown bear in Katmai National Park, Alaska, with partially eaten salmon.

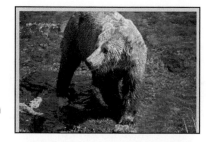

▪ Some chimpanzees use tools to help obtain food.

▪ In Japanese culture it is very polite to bow to another person when meeting them. At the Nara Temple near Osaka, Japan, many of the Sika deer that live around the temple have learnt that they are more likely to be given some food if they bow their head to a person.

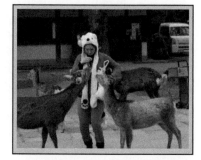

4.7 Sika deer at the Nara Temple.

▪ Vervet monkeys have three different warning calls – leopard, snake and eagle. The young have to learn what type of response to make to each call. They also have to learn how to distinguish between an eagle (predator) and a vulture (harmless).

▪ In dense African forest visual communication is difficult. Mongooses and several species of monkey hunt together and respond to each other's warning calls. In this way there is a lookout at all levels from ground to canopy.

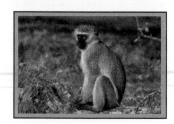

4.8 Vervet monkey.

▪ Young elephants will learn from the matriarch of the herd where to find water during the dry season.

Learning in Humans

❖ **Key points**

➢ Compared to all other animals humans have the greatest capacity for learning and have an extended childhood with parental care to make use of this. Motor skills such as talking, walking, writing or playing a musical instrument all require learning. Much learning is done by watching and listening to older people.
➢ For example, Australian aboriginal people teach their children to recognize specific trees or rock formations in order to navigate around their lands to find food, water and shelter.
➢ Learning starts early in childhood and continues through to old age.

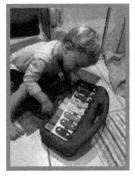

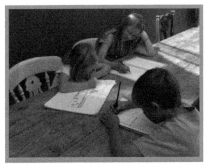

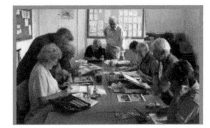

4.11 Older people studying at the North Wiltshire Branch of the University of the Third Age in the UK.

4.10 Children at different stages of learning.

4.9 A baby playing with a toy piano.

Example of data analysis of invertebrate behaviour

➢ Woodlice are terrestrial crustaceans that breathe through gills and therefore require a damp environment.
➢ They are predated upon by birds so hide during the day.
➢ If placed in a choice chamber in the dark with one side damp and the other side dry they will tend to settle in the damp side.
➢ Data can be collected and statistically analysed using the chi squared test – see Core Guide HL *page 11*.

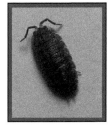

4.12 A woodlouse

Trial	Dry	Wet
1	2	8
2	1	9
3	3	7
4	3	7
5	2	8
Total	11	39

Classes	Observed O	Expected E	O - E	$(O - E)^2$	$\dfrac{(O - E)^2}{E}$
Dry	11	25	-14	196	7.84
Wet	39	25	+14	196	7,84
Totals	50	50	0		$\Sigma = 15.68$

The null hypothesis states that woodlice have no preference for the wet or dry side.
At the 5% level this result is highly significant, disproving the null hypothesis.

1. List four characteristics of innate behaviour.

2. Which type of neuron links sensory and motor neurons in the spinal cord?

3. Through which root do motor neurons leave the spinal cord?

4. Name two types of effector.

5. Which part of the nervous system controls reflexes?

6. Label the diagram in the 9 places indicated.

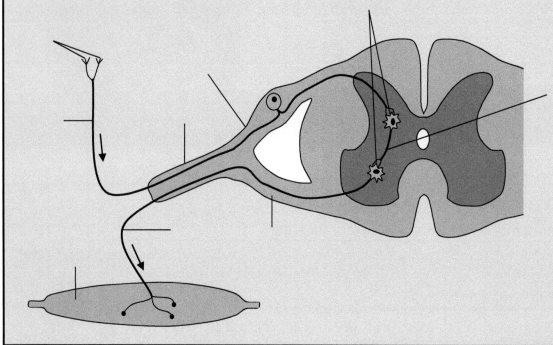

7a. Which type of behaviour requires memory?

7b. This type of behaviour develops as a result of experience. List two sources of this experience.

8. What is reflex conditioning?

9. Outline Pavlov's reflex conditioning experiment.

10. What is operant conditioning?

11. Outline Skinner's operant conditioning experiment.

12. What is imprinting?

13. Outline Lorenz's imprinting experiment.

IB Option A © Ashby Merson-Davies

Self-test quiz

1. Which of the following statements about innate behaviour is correct?
   a. It is genetically controlled and therefore inherited from parents.
   b. It is a set of behaviour patterns determined by the changing environmental conditions.
   c. It only appears in young animals as a result of being looked after by parents for a long time.
   d. It is a type of behaviour that develops as an animal gets older and more experienced.

2. Which of the following is the correct pathway for a reflex action?
   a. Receptor – motor neuron – relay neuron – sensory neuron – effector.
   b. Receptor – sensory neuron – relay neuron – motor neuron – effector.
   c. Effector – motor neuron – relay neuron – sensory neuron – receptor.
   d. Receptor – relay neuron – sensory neuron – motor neuron – effector.

3. Which of the following is a correct statement about effectors?
   a. They are only secretory glands.
   b. They are only muscles.
   c. They are endocrine glands, exocrine glands and muscles.
   d. They are only the glands that secrete hormones.

4. Which of the following statements about learned behaviour is correct?
   a. It is passed from parent to offspring through DNA.
   b. It can only be acquired as a result of offspring watching their parents' behaviour.
   c. It is a behaviour pattern acquired as a result of environmental experiences.
   d. It is a behaviour pattern involving a number of reflex actions.

5. Which of the following is a correct description of reflex conditioning?
   a. It is a behavioural response only shown by dogs.
   b. It is a response which involves developing new associations.
   c. It is a learned response to help survival.
   d. It is a response to a stimulus which requires memory.

6. Which of the following is a correct description of operant conditioning?
   a. It is an automatic response to a stimulus.
   b. It is a condition which operates through a series of reflexes.
   c. It is a response only shown by caged animals.
   d. It is a response to a stimulus which requires memory.

7. Certain species of songbird develop their song by modifying an innate song pattern after listening to adult birds singing. This is called:
   a. Imprinting.
   b. Latent learning.
   c. Operant learning.
   d. Adolescent juvenile learning

A5 Neuropharmacology

Neurotransmitters and Synapses

❖ **Key points**

➢ Synapses are junctions between neurons. (*Revise* Core Guide HL *page 167*).
➢ Each neuron has many synapses with other neurons.
➢ The neurotransmitters in these synapses can have an inhibitory or excitatory effect.
➢ An action potential in the post synaptic neuron will only occur if the potential difference at the **axon hillock** rises above the value of the threshold potential.
➢ Impulses arriving through excitatory and inhibitory neurons will summate – *see examples below*.

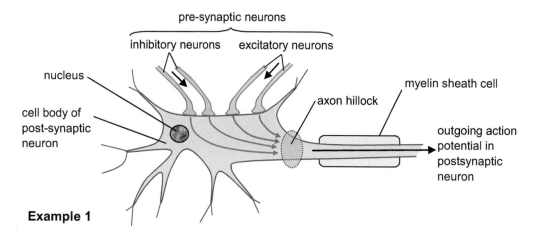

Example 1

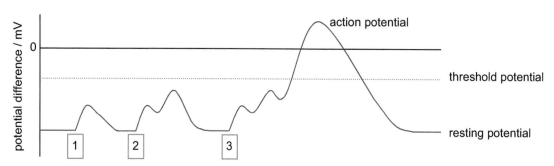

1 An impulse arrives through an excitatory neuron but the rise in potential difference is insufficient to reach the threshold and so an action potential does not occur.

2 Two excitatory impulses arrive close together and add up, (summation), but are still unable to reach the threshold and so an action potential does not occur.

3 Three presynaptic impulses arrive close together and add up, and this time do reach the threshold so an action potential does occur.

The neurotransmitter itself is neither excitatory nor inhibitory. It simply activates a receptor on the postsynaptic membrane and it is this receptor that determines the effect.

Excitatory: - the receptor opens a channel that allows positive ions (Na^+ or K^+) to diffuse <u>into</u> the postsynaptic neuron which raises the resting potential closer to the threshold.

Inhibitory: - the receptor opens a channel that either allows negative ions (Cl^-) to diffuse <u>into</u> the postsynaptic neuron, or allows positive ions (K^+) to diffuse <u>out of</u> the postsynaptic neuron. Both of these actions lower the resting potential further from the threshold.

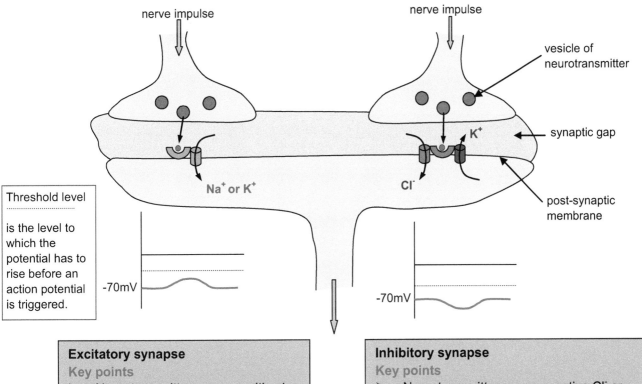

Threshold level

is the level to which the potential has to rise before an action potential is triggered.

Excitatory synapse

Key points

➢ Neurotransmitter opens positive ion channels on post-synaptic membrane.
➢ Resting potential raised closer to threshold level for post-synaptic potential to be triggered.
➢ This enhances the probability of depolarisation.

Inhibitory synapse

Key points

➢ Neurotransmitter opens negative Cl⁻ or positive K⁺ channels on post-synaptic membrane.
➢ Resting potential lowered further from threshold level for post-synaptic potential to be triggered.
➢ This reduces the probability of depolarisation.
➢ (This is called hyperpolarisation.)

Example 2

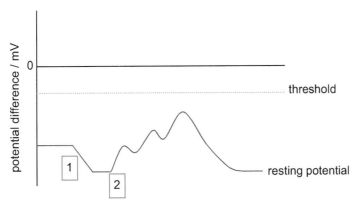

1 │ An impulse arrives through an inhibitory neuron and this makes the resting potential more negative, about -80mV. Note that the threshold value does not change.

2 │ The three rapid impulses that in the first diagram caused an action potential now have no effect as the threshold is not reached.

➢ Decisions are made by these multiple synapses.
➢ The effect of all the incoming impulses is **summated** at the axon hillock and if the threshold is reached then an action potential in the postsynaptic neuron is produced.

- To illustrate this assume a value of at least +3 is required to initiate an action potential.
- Each inhibitory impulse contributes -1 at the axon hillock.
- Each excitatory impulse contributes +1 at the axon hillock.

Example	Inhibitory impulses	Excitatory impulses	Net value at axon hillock	Action potential
1	0	2	+2	no
2	1	4	+3	yes
3	2	4	+2	no
4	2	6	+4	yes

Slow-acting neurotransmitters

❖ **Key points**

➤ There are many different neurotransmitters acting in the brain.

➤ Some of these such as glutamate (excitatory) and gamma-aminobutyric acid (GABA) (inhibitory) are fast acting, affecting a post synaptic potential within one millisecond.

> Glutamate is excitatory because it opens Na^+ channels; GABA is inhibitory because it opens Cl^- channels – see previous page.

➤ This is done by opening ion channels.

➤ Other neurotransmitters, such as dopamine, norepinephrine and serotonin, are slow acting, taking hundreds of milliseconds to minutes to have an effect.

➤ They bind to different post synaptic receptors and trigger a cascade of events, including protein synthesis via a second messenger pathway.

➤ These proteins could be enzymes, receptors or channel proteins.

➤ This results in:
- An increase in the number of neurotransmitter vesicles in the presynaptic region.
- An increase in the number of neurotransmitter receptors on the postsynaptic membrane.

➤ Their role is to modulate (regulate/adjust) the functioning of the fast acting synapses through these proteins.

➤ They can also leave the synapse and diffuse through the surrounding tissue fluid to affect other neurons or groups of neurons.

➤ Their effect can last for days thus affecting the actual post synaptic output produced by further release of fast acting neurotransmitters.

➤ This is called long term potentiation (LTP).

Memory and learning

❖ **Key points**

➤ This is due to synaptic plasticity – the ability of synapses to strengthen or weaken over time in response to increases or decreases in their activity.

➤ It involves both long term potentiation (LTP) and long term depression (LTD).

➤ A synaptic pathway used frequently will become stronger through the action of slow acting neurotransmitters – LTP.

➤ This is the process of learning – repeating something, such as a list of the vocabulary required for DNA replication.

➤ The more often it is repeated the stronger the memory.

➤ If a pathway is used less often then it needs to be 'cleaned up' by removal of neurotransmitter vesicles and receptors.

➤ This is LTD.

➤ It creates space for the components used for strengthening a pathway.

Psychoactive drugs – the brain and personality

❖ **Key points**

- Drugs are chemicals which enter the body by breathing, injection, or eaten.
- They affect synaptic transmission in the brain.
- The effect can stimulate (excitatory) or depress (inhibitory) postsynaptic transmission.
- Stimulant drugs mimic the stimulation provided by the sympathetic nervous system – see page 8.

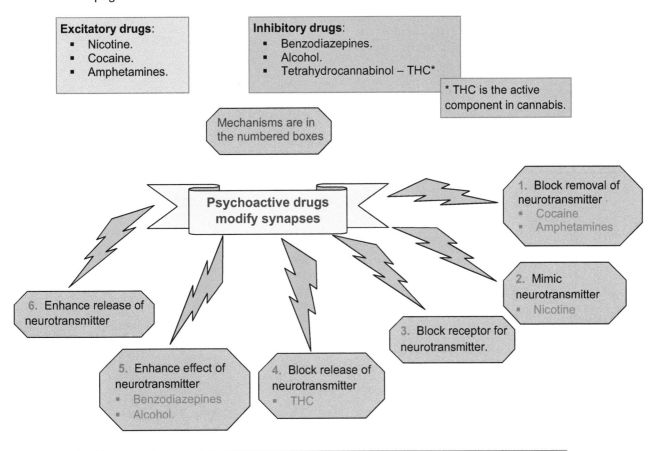

Excitatory drugs:
- Nicotine.
- Cocaine.
- Amphetamines.

Inhibitory drugs:
- Benzodiazepines.
- Alcohol.
- Tetrahydrocannabinol – THC*

* THC is the active component in cannabis.

Mechanisms are in the numbered boxes

Psychoactive drugs modify synapses

1. Block removal of neurotransmitter
   - Cocaine
   - Amphetamines

2. Mimic neurotransmitter
   - Nicotine

3. Block receptor for neurotransmitter.

4. Block release of neurotransmitter
   - THC

5. Enhance effect of neurotransmitter
   - Benzodiazepines
   - Alcohol.

6. Enhance release of neurotransmitter

The actual effect is determined by whether the synapse is excitatory or inhibitory.

Drug action	Synapse	Result
Blocks	Excitatory	Depression
Enhances	Excitatory	Stimulation
Blocks	Inhibitory	Stimulation
Enhances	Inhibitory	Depression

Six examples of drugs are given below. You need to know two from each column.

| Stimulants | Sedatives |

Cocaine
- Source - leaves of the coca bush that grows in the Andes.
- Mechanism type 1 at dopaminergic synapses. (Reduces activity of the gene that makes the receptor.)
- Effects - Dopamine remains in synaptic gap. Increased energy and alertness; more talkative; constricts blood vessels; elevates body temperature; increases heart rate and blood pressure; increases pleasure feelings.
- Crack is a form of cocaine that can be heated to form a vapour. This is rapidly absorbed through the nasal capillaries; gives intense feelings of euphoria.
- Highly addictive. Gradually body makes less dopamine and so becomes dependent on presence of cocaine.

Nicotine
- Source - tobacco leaves.
- Mechanism type 2 at cholinergic synapses, except those in heart muscle.
- Effects – Stimulates transmission in many parts of the brain.
- Strongly addictive.

Amphetamines
- Source – Prescription drugs such as Ritalin. 'Street' drugs such as Ecstasy (methylenedioxymethamphetamine).
- Mechanism type 1 at dopaminergic synapses.
- Effects – increased alertness, euphoria, increased pulse rate and blood pressure, insomnia, loss of appetite. May increase body temperature and cause hallucinations and convulsions.
- High potential for psychological dependence.

Tetrahydrocannabinol – THC
- Source – Hemp plant (Marijuana).
- Active ingredient is a compound called THC.
- Mechanism type 4 by blocking fusing of neurotransmitter vesicles with pre-synaptic membrane.
- It does this by inhibiting the uptake of Ca^{2+} through the presynaptic membrane – see page 167 of the Core Guide.
- Effects – Euphoria; relaxed inhibitions; increased appetite; dulling of pain; in higher doses produce psychedelic effects; may cause panic and paranoia; may interfere with learning and memory.
- May result in some psychological dependence.

Alcohol
- Source – wide range of drinks.
- Mechanism type 5 at GABA synapses. GABA (gamma aminobutyric acid) is the neurotransmitter at inhibitory synapses in the brain. Alcohol binds to a site on the post-synaptic receptor different from the GABA binding site and enhances the strength of GABA binding. Thus more Cl^- is allowed in and the synapse is hyperpolarised.
- Similar to benzodiazepines.
- Effects - Lower doses relaxes inhibitions, reduces reaction time, hence it is dangerous to drive; higher doses causes loss of memory, loss of co-ordination and unconsciousness; may produce violent behaviour.
- Can result in addiction.

Benzodiazepines
- Source – Prescription anti-anxiety drugs such as Valium and Librion.
- Mechanism type 5 at GABA synapses. GABA (gamma aminobutyric acid) is the neurotransmitter at inhibitory synapses in the brain. Drug binds to a site on the post-synaptic receptor different from the GABA binding site and enhances the strength of GABA binding. Thus more Cl^- is allowed in and the synapse is hyperpolarised – see page 33.
- Similar to alcohol.
- Effects - Lower doses reduces anxiety; higher doses produces disorientation and drunken behaviour.
- May result in some psychological dependence.

Addiction

❖ Points for discussion

Dopamine secretion:
- Dopamine affects brain processes that control emotional response and feelings of pleasure.
- Thus anything that increases activity at dopamine synapses, and hence the feelings of pleasure, is likely to be repeated.

Social factors:
- These can play a key role.
- Drugs may provide an 'escape' from poverty and social deprivation.
- Peer pressure.
- Cultural: used in a religious or shamanic context.
- People with mental health problems.

Genetic predisposition:
- Susceptibility to drugs of any sort – nicotine, sleeping tablets, anti-depressants, psychoactive drugs - varies from person to person.
- Desensitisation to a drug, i.e. the effect from the same sized dose gets less and less, can take a long time in some people and in others a single dose is sufficient.
- There appear to be family traits.
- The above points both imply a genetic component.
- Further research needs to be done to identify the genes involved.
- Results from the Human Genome Project may assist with this.

Anaesthetics

❖ Key points

- Local anaesthetics act by interfering with neural transmission between areas of sensory perception and the CNS.
- They work by preventing the sodium voltage gated channels from opening and so preventing the transmission of nerve impulses from the pain receptors– *see* Core Guide SL *page 126*, HL *page 165*.
- The patient is fully conscious and is aware of what is going on but cannot feel pain.
- Example – Lidocaine is a local anaesthetic used in dentistry.
  - General anaesthetics cause the patient to become unconscious and therefore totally unaware.
  - They would be used for delicate surgery where the patient must not move, or for major surgery.
  - They are most commonly injected into a vein in the back of the hand.
- Example – Propofol.
  - An epidural anaesthetic is often used in childbirth.
  - It is injected into the epidural space, which is a space between the vertebra and the spinal cord.
  - This blocks sensory pain nerves that enter the spinal cord.
  - The patient is fully conscious and is aware of what is going on but cannot feel pain.

Endorphins

❖ Key points

- Pain receptors are distributed through most parts of the body.
- They detect chemicals, such as those in a wasp sting or snake bite, punctures of the skin such as by a thorn, or excess heat.
- Sensory neurons carry signals from the receptors to sensory areas of the cerebral cortex which give the sensation of pain.
- Endorphins are neurotransmitters secreted by the anterior pituitary gland, hypothalamus, spinal cord and specific regions of the brain.
- They bind to opioid receptors at sensory synapses in the peripheral nervous system.
- This leads to preventing the release of substance P, a key protein involved in the transmission of pain.

1. What is meant by the threshold value for a synapse?

2. State the two types of neuron that can form synapses.

3. State two ways that an inhibitory neurotransmitter works.

4. State an example of a slow-acting neurotransmitter.

5. Approximately how long does it take for a slow-acting neurotransmitter to have an effect?

6. What is meant by the term summation?

7. Distinguish between the action of fast-acting and slow-acting neurotransmitters.

8. What is synaptic plasticity?

11a. State two examples of excitatory (stimulant) psychoactive drugs.

11b. Using one of your examples state how it affects synaptic transmission.

12a. State two examples of inhibitory (sedative) psychoactive drugs.

12b. Using one of your examples state how it affects synaptic transmission.

13. State why dopamine secretion may lead to addiction.

14. List the social factors that may lead to addiction.

15. Apart from social factors what other factor may lead to drug addiction?

16. How does a local anaesthetic work?

17. Distinguish between awareness for local and general anaesthetics.

Self-test quiz

1. Which of the following statements about synapses is correct?
   a. An excitatory impulse arriving on the presynaptic side always results in an impulse from the postsynaptic side.
   b. An inhibitory impulse at a synapse raises the action potential in the postsynaptic neuron by allowing sodium ions to flow in.
   c. A postsynaptic output is determined by the interaction between excitatory and inhibitory synaptic inputs.
   d. Excitatory impulses at a synapse cause the release of chloride ions into the postsynaptic neuron which lowers the threshold value.

2. Which of the following statements about the threshold value of a synapse is correct?
   a. It is the level of depolarisation that must be reached before a postsynaptic potential can be triggered.
   b. It is the result of summation of excitatory impulses arriving at the presynaptic region.
   c. It is the level of depolarisation that occurs in the postsynaptic region.
   d. It is a value of 0mV inside the presynaptic region.

3. Which of the following statements about neurotransmitters is correct?
   a. Fast-acting neurotransmitters can be both excitatory and inhibitory.
   b. Fast-acting neurotransmitters are always excitatory.
   c. Slow-acting neurotransmitters are always inhibitory.
   d. Fast-acting neurotransmitters work only at particular synapses and slow-acting neurotransmitters only work at other synapses.

4. Which of the following statements about synaptic plasticity is correct?
   a. The number of synapses formed during development of the brain remains constant.
   b. Synaptic plasticity is the ability of a synapse to change its threshold potential.
   c. Synaptic plasticity is a change to a synapse brought about by fast-acting excitatory neurotransmitters.
   d. The number of synapses on the cell body of a neuron can be changed depending on how the synapses are used.

5. Which of the following statements about memory and learning is correct?
   a. It results from changes to the type of neurotransmitter used at a synapse.
   b. It involves slow-acting neurotransmitters.
   c. It requires the growth of new axons.
   d. It involves fast-acting neurotransmitters modifying the actions of slow-acting neurotransmitters.

6. Which line in the table is correct?

	Excitatory drugs	Inhibitory drugs
a.	Nicotine; amphetamines; tetrahydrocannabinol.	Benzodiazepines; alcohol; cocaine.
b.	Amphetamines; tetrahydrocannabinol; alcohol.	Benzodiazepines; nicotine; cocaine.
c.	Nicotine; cocaine; amphetamines.	Benzodiazepines; alcohol; tetrahydrocannabinol.
d.	Benzodiazepines; alcohol; tetrahydrocannabinol.	Nicotine; cocaine; amphetamines.

7. Which of the following statements about addiction is <u>not</u> true?
   a. Some people are more susceptible to addiction because there is a genetic component.
   b. A particular drug always has the same effect in different people.
   c. Repeatedly taking a drug brings about desensitisation meaning more is required to have the same effect.
   d. Drug taking can result from peer pressure in gangs.

8. Which of the following statements about anaesthetics is correct?
   a. They prevent pain receptors in the skin from depolarising.
   b. They block transmission of nerve impulses in motor neurons leading to the CNS.
   c. They prevent the release of neurotransmitters at pain synapses between sensory and relay neurons in the spinal cord.
   d. They vary in the level of awareness experienced by a patient.

A6 Ethology

> Ethology is the study of animal behaviour in natural conditions.

❖ **Key points**

➢ Natural selection can change the frequency of observed animal behaviour.
➢ Behaviour that increases the chances of survival and reproduction will become more common in a population; learned behaviour can spread through a population or be lost from it more rapidly than innate behaviour.

Migratory behaviour – Blackcap (*Sylvia atricapilla*)

❖ **Key points**

6.1 The Eurasian Blackcap (*Sylvia atricapilla*)

Migration is movement over long distances.
➢ Breeds over most of Europe.
➢ German blackcaps normally migrate southwest to over-winter in Spain. ⟶
➢ Rising winter temperatures in the UK increased food supplies.
➢ More birds are now found in the UK during the winter months but ringing studies show that they bred in Germany. ⟶
➢ Over-wintering birds were captured in the UK and Spain, taken to Germany and bred over two seasons.
➢ Thus all birds had the same environmental cues.
➢ Observations on migration behaviour in captivity showed the birds would fly in a direction that took them to their expected over-wintering region.
➢ This shows that the direction of migration is genetically programmed.
➢ Birds that do not fly as far south to over-winter can get back to the breeding grounds sooner and with less expenditure of energy.
➢ This will give them a selective advantage over those birds that have to return from further south.
➢ Birds from Austria tended to fly southeast to the eastern Mediterranean and then south to over-winter in eastern Africa. ⟶
➢ Cross-breeding the Austrian and German birds produced offspring that tended to fly in a direction between those of the parent populations. ⋯⟶
➢ This is further evidence that migration direction is genetically controlled.

Autumn migration routes of the Blackcap.

Altruistic behaviour – Vampire bat (*Desmodus rotundus*)

❖ **Key points**

➢ Found in Central and South America.
➢ Form social groups, colonies, of unrelated individuals.
➢ Nocturnal feeders on fresh blood from animals such as horses and cattle.
➢ The chance of failing to feed successfully is quite high.
➢ Bats failing to find food on two consecutive nights usually die of starvation.
➢ If a bat returns to the colony hungry other, unrelated bats feed it.
➢ A bat that has been fed in this way will give food at another time.
➢ Because the risk of failing to feed is quite high it is beneficial for a well fed bat to give food to a hungry bat since another time it may fail to feed and could die if it did not receive food from another bat.
➢ This is called **reciprocal altruism**.
➢ An important difference with the Florida Scrub Jay (see Additional Examples on page 44) is that the individuals involved may not be genetically related.

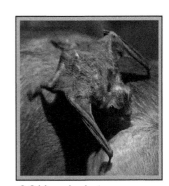

6.2 Vampire bat, (*Desmodus rotundus*)

Foraging behaviour – Shore crab (*Carcinus maenas*)

❖ **Key points**
➢ Foraging behaviour is searching for food.
➢ The shore crab feeds on mussels.
➢ For a given sized crab there is an optimal mussel size for which prey value is at a maximum.
➢ Prey value is the ratio between energy content and handling time.
➢ Handling time is the time taken to open the mussel.
➢ The larger the mussel the greater the energy content but the greater the time taken and energy expenditure in opening the mussel.
➢ Given a wide choice of mussel sizes the crabs select the optimal size, i.e. the size that gives the greatest energy content relative to the energy spent in gaining it.
➢ Suboptimal mussels will be selected if encountered frequently even if there is an abundance of optimal ones.
➢ This is because it is more profitable to gain less energy from a suboptimal mussel rather than expend energy searching for an optimal one.

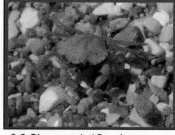

6.3 Shore crab (*Carcinus maenas*)

Breeding strategies – Coho salmon (*Oncorhynchus kisutch*)

❖ **Key points**

➢ Coho salmon live in the North Pacific Ocean but breed in rivers.
➢ The females release their eggs and a male then releases sperm over the eggs.
➢ The breeding males are in two forms – hooknoses and jacks.
➢ **Hooknoses:**
  • Grow slowly and return to the rivers to breed after three years.
  • They are large and brightly coloured.
  • They fight other hooknoses for access to a female laying eggs.
➢ **Jacks:**
  • Grow quickly and return to the rivers to breed after two years.
  • They are smaller, less brightly coloured and cannot fight the hooknoses.
  • They try and remain hidden and then sneak up on a female laying eggs.
➢ It would seem that the jacks are at a reproductive disadvantage since they are likely to be seen by hooknoses and chased away.
➢ However it has been shown that jacks produce more sperm and higher quality sperm than hooknoses which increases the probability of their sperm fertilising the eggs.
➢ Jacks invest more energy into larger testes and improved sperm quality rather than larger body size.

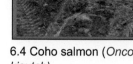

6.4 Coho salmon (*Oncorhynchus kisutch*)

Courtship behaviour – Birds of Paradise

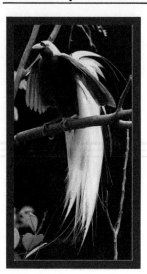

❖ **Key points**

➢ Birds of paradise, found on the island of New Guinea, show extremes of exaggerated traits.
➢ Only the males show these traits.
➢ The bright feathers and displays make the birds very obvious to predators, could hinder their escape and make searching for food more difficult.
➢ Thus an individual that is in good condition and able to display is likely to be very strong.
➢ These characteristics would be genetically determined.
➢ A female selecting such an individual is therefore selecting strong genes.
➢ The females must also have genes that select for these exaggerated traits.

6.5 The Lesser bird of paradise (*Paradisaea minor*)

IB Option A © Ashby Merson-Davies

Synchronised oestrous – Lion (*Panthera leo*)

❖ **Key points**

➢ Oestrus is the time in the oestrous cycle when female mammals become receptive to males and fertilisation is likely to occur after mating.

➢ Lions live in small groups called prides consisting of several lionesses and a single male.

➢ The lionesses do the hunting and so it is beneficial for them all to have their cubs at the same time.

➢ This allows one lioness to look after the cubs while the others are hunting.

➢ A lioness will suckle cubs that are not hers.

➢ The male remains close by to help protect the cubs.

➢ This increases the chances of survival of the cubs.

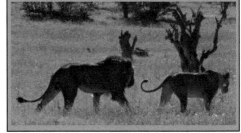

6.6 A pair of lions (*Panthera leo*) in Etosha National Park, Namibia.

Development and loss of learned behaviour – Blue tit (*Cyanistes caeruleus*)

❖ **Key points**

➢ The blue tit is a small bird common in Europe.

➢ In the UK and other European countries at the beginning of the 20th century milk began to be delivered to households early in the morning, with the milkman simply filling jugs left on the doorstep.

➢ The milk was always full cream and the cream floats on the top.

➢ Blue tits quickly learned this was a rich source of food, especially in the winter.

➢ During the 1920's the milk began to be delivered in bottles that had aluminium foil tops.

➢ Blue tits quickly learned that they could peck through the thin foil cap to get at the cream.

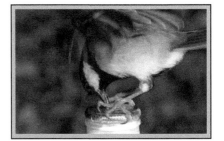

6.7 A blue tit (*Cyanistes caeruleus*) pecking at a milk bottle top.

➢ Blue tits are quite social birds and in the winter feed together in groups of up to 10 birds.

➢ Thus this learned behaviour was able to spread quickly.

➢ This method of milk delivery gradually decreased due to the cost of the service, milk becoming available in larger plastic bottles in supermarkets and the change of people's preference to skimmed or semi-skimmed milk.

➢ The blue tits that had learned to peck at bottles quickly lost this behaviour pattern.

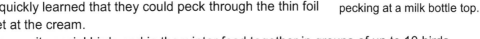

A few European robins (*Erithacus rubecula*) also learnt this behaviour but they are territorial birds and do not form groups. This behaviour therefore did not spread and quickly died out.

Additional Examples

The syllabus states that other examples should be studied if possible, so here are three more for you to look at.

Florida scrub jay (*Aphelocoma coerulescens*)

Altruistic behaviour

❖ **Key points**

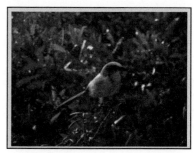

6.8 Florida scrub jay (*Aphelocoma coerulescens*)

➢ This is a bird found in the drier shrub areas of Florida.
➢ Shows altruistic behaviour for a short time.
➢ Offspring of a pair from the previous breeding season help to feed the next brood, defend the territory and watch for predators.
➢ They remain non-reproductive till next breeding season.
➢ Nests with helpers have more offspring than those that don't.
➢ Helpers share genes with new brood so being altruistic increases chances of shared genes passing to later generations.

Bluegill fish (*Lepomis macrochirus*) feeding on Daphnia

Foraging behaviour

❖ **Key points**

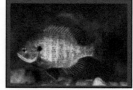

6.9 Bluegill fish (*Lepomis macrochirus*)   6.10 Daphnia

➢ Daphnia are small fresh water crustaceans that are born fully formed and grow larger.
➢ This gives the fish a choice of sizes.
➢ At low Daphnia numbers the fish eat all sizes in order to gain enough energy.
➢ As Daphnia numbers increase the fish become more and more selective and eat an increasing proportion of the larger ones.
➢ This optimises the energy intake for the energy expenditure.

Oystercatchers (*Haematopus ostralegus*) feeding on limpets (*Patella* sp.)

Foraging behaviour

❖ **Key points**

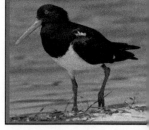

6.11 Oystercatcher (*Haematopus ostralegus*)

➢ Limpets inhabit rocky shores and when covered by water graze on algae.
➢ As the tide goes out the limpets return to their home site which is shaped to fit their shell.
➢ They prevent desiccation by clamping onto the rock; they can be solitary or rest in clusters.
➢ It was found that oystercatchers preferred to attack solitary limpets rather than those in clusters.
➢ There was no nutritional or size difference between solitary and clustered limpets.
➢ Oystercatchers preferred to attack the anterior end of the limpet.

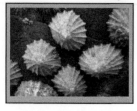

6.12 Limpets (*Patella* sp.)

➢ This anterior end was more exposed to the angle of attack in a solitary limpet because when clustered neighbouring limpets often prevented this preferred attack angle.
➢ When one limpet in a cluster was attacked the other limpets responded by clamping down more tightly making it very difficult for the oystercatcher to remove them.
➢ Thus the oystercatcher expended less energy by attacking solitary limpets.

   IB Option A © Ashby Merson-Davies

1. What is the name given to the study of animals in natural conditions?	2. What is the value of behaviour that increases the chance of survival?

3. Blackcaps that were overwintering in Spain and England were captured and during the summer were allowed to breed in separate aviaries next to each other in their normal breeding grounds in Germany. In the autumn they were observed to determine in which direction they would fly to overwinter. Those birds collected in England showed a flight pattern towards England and those collected in Spain showed a flight pattern towards Spain.
What does this indicate about the control of the migratory behaviour?

4. If a vampire bat is unsuccessful at getting a meal when it returns to the roost is likely to be given some food by a bat that did feed. What is the name given to this type of behaviour?	5. What is the benefit to lions of synchronised oestrus?

6. When milk was delivered to doorsteps in foil-capped milk bottles birds called blue tits pecked through the caps to drink the cream. Give two reasons why this was considered to be learned behaviour and not innate.

Self-test quiz

1. Which of the following is the correct description of ethology?
   a. The study of the behaviour of animals in natural conditions.
   b. The study of the behaviour of animals in zoos and laboratories.
   c. Comparisons of behaviour of wild animals with captive animals.
   d. The study of the behaviour of wild animals adapting to captive conditions.

2. Which line in the table is the correct term for the description in the column headings?

	Shore crabs searching for mussels on a rocky beach	Vampire bats sharing a blood meal at the roost during the day.	A Blackcap flying from its breeding grounds in Germany to its overwintering grounds in Spain.
a.	Altruistic behaviour	Foraging behaviour	Migratory behaviour
b.	Foraging behaviour	Altruistic behaviour	Breeding strategy
c.	Migratory behaviour	Breeding strategy	Foraging behaviour
d.	Foraging behaviour	Altruistic behaviour	Migratory behaviour

3. Birds of Paradise are found only on the island of New Guinea. The males have extravagant plumage and courtship displays. The females watch these displays. The best term to describe this is:
   a. Mating behaviour.
   b. Mate selection.
   c. Showing off.
   d. Display behaviour.

4. Lions (*Panthera leo*) live in small groups called prides consisting of several lionesses and a single male. The lionesses synchronise oestrus. The purpose of this is:
   a. Because it makes it easier for the male to mate with the females.
   b. The females do not have to fight each other in order to mate with the male.
   c. It encourages the male to hunt for food.
   d. the cubs are born to all the females at the same time.

Appendix

Glossary

Apoptosis	Programmed cell death.
Dopaminergic synapse	A synapse which uses dopamine as the neurotransmitter.
Shamanic	This is a practice that involves a practitioner reaching altered states of consciousness in order to perceive and interact with a spirit world and channel these transcendental energies into this world.

Answers to Grey Box Questions

Underlined words are required.

A1
1. Neural plate.
2. Neural crest.
3. Dendron / dendrite.
4. Axon.
5. Another neuron; a muscle.
6. Neural pruning; apoptosis / programmed cell death.
7. Repeated use.
8. Spina bifida.
9. Damage to a part of the brain.
10. Blockage / blood clot in blood supply; burst blood vessel.

A2
1. See diagram on page 7.
2. Neural plate.
3. It becomes folded.
4. Breathing; heart rate; swallowing; gut muscles; blood vessels.
5. Speech.
6. Pleasure / reward centre.
7. Occipital lobe.
8. A graph showing the electrical activity of the brain.
9. A light shone into the eye causes the pupil diameter to decrease.
10. Medulla (oblongata).
11. Relating any changes in behaviour to the affected part of the brain.
12. Dissection / examination after death.
13. An fMRI can detect an increase in the flow of blood when a part of the brain becomes active.
14. Animal experimentation.
15. Positive.

A3
1. See page 15.
2. Cone.
3. Rod.
4. Cone.
5. Right.
6. Three.
7. Abnormal photopigment in the red of green cones / loss of red or green cones.
8. See page 15.
9. See page 16.
10. See page 20.
11. See page 20
12. Pinna.
13. Transfer the vibrations of the ear drum to the oval window.
14. To allow movements of the oval window / moves out when the oval window moves in.
15. Movement of the oval window causes movement of the fluid in the cochlea which moves sensory hairs which send nerve impulses to the brain.
16. Semi-circular canals.

A4
1. Inherited; develops independently from the environment; occurs in all members of the species; is in the form of reflexes.
2. Relay neuron.
3. Ventral root.
4. Endocrine gland; muscle.
5. Autonomic nervous system.
6. See page 25.
7a. Learned behaviour.
7b. Environment / observing another individual / parent.
8. The modification of behaviour in an animal in response to a repeated stimulus such that the stimulus and response become associated.
9. See page 26
10. A learning mechanism in which the reward follows only after the correct behavioural response.
11. See page 26
12. An attachment to an object encountered during a sensitive time period, often immediately after birth.
13. See page 27.

A5

1. The minimum potential that has to be reached before an action potential is reached / a post synaptic impulse is generated.
2. Excitatory and inhibitory.
3. Causes K^+ ions to diffuse into the synaptic gap/cleft; causes Cl^- ions to diffuse out of the synaptic gap.
4. Dopamine / norepinephrine/serotonin.
5. Hundreds of milliseconds to minutes.
6. The effect of each incoming nerve impulse is added.
7. See page 34
8. The ability of synapses to strengthen or weaken over time in response to increases or decreases in their activity.
9. Learning involves repeated uses of synapses which strengthens them.
10. The synapse is inhibited / depression.
11a. Nicotine / cocaine / amphetamines.   11b. See page 35
12a. Benzodiazepines / alcohol / tetrahydrocannabinol – THC.   12b.   See page 35
13. It stimulates the pleasure centres of the brain.
14. Drugs may provide an 'escape' from poverty and social deprivation.
    Peer pressure in 'gangs'.
    Cultural - used in a religious or shamanic context.
    People with mental health problems.
15. Genetic predisposition.
16. Prevent the voltage gated sodium channels from opening.
17. Local – fully conscious but cannot feel any sensation from the area being operated on.
    General – unconscious and unaware of any sensation.

A6

1. Ethology.   2.   Increases the chances of reproduction / passing on genes to offspring.
3. It is genetically controlled.   4.   Altruism.
5. All the cubs are born at the same time.
6. It spread from region to region.
   The behaviour was quickly lost when people changed to semi-skimmed or skimmed milk / milk was delivered in plastic capped bottles / doorstep deliveries decreased.

Answers to Self-test quizzes

Question	A1	A2	A3	A4	A5	A6
1	c	b	b	a	c	a
2	a	a	b	b	a	d
3	d	d	c	c	a	b
4	c	b	a	c	d	d
5	b	a	d	b	b	
6		b	c	d	c	
7		c	b	b	b	
8		a	b		d	
9		d	a			
10		b	c			
11			b			

Acknowledgements

1.1. © Corrian Homan Design Studio.

1.2. © Nrets at en.wikipedia (Transferred from en.wikipedia) [CC BY 2.5 (http://creativecommons.org/licenses/by/2.5)], via Wikimedia Commons.

1.3 © Hellerhoff (Own work) [CC BY-SA 3.0 (http://creativecommons.org/licenses/by-sa/3.0) or GFDL (http://www.gnu.org/copyleft/fdl.html)], via Wikimedia Commons

1.4 © Centers for Disease Control and Prevention (Centers for Disease Control and Prevention) [CC0], via Wikimedia Commons

1.5 © Lucien Monfils (Own work) [GFDL (http://www.gnu.org/copyleft/fdl.html) or CC BY-SA 3.0 (http://creativecommons.org/licenses/by-sa/3.0)], via Wikimedia Commons

2.1, 2.3, 2.4, 2.5 © Shutterstock

2.2 © Polygon data were generated by Database Center for Life Science(DBCLS)[2]. (Polygon data are from BodyParts3D[1]) [CC BY-SA 2.1 jp (http://creativecommons.org/licenses/by-sa/2.1/jp/deed.en)], via Wikimedia Commons

2.6 © Thuglas at en.wikipedia [Public domain], from Wikimedia Commons

2.7 © Dr. Al Jenny [Public domain], via Wikimedia Commons

2.8 Image courtesy of Steve Smith, FMRI Centre, Department of Clinical Neurology, University of Oxford.

2.9 © Dr. Johannes Sobotta [Public domain], via Wikimedia Commons

3.1 Photo courtesy of Neil Donnelly, Eyelines Opticians, Sevenoaks, UK

3.2 © Mark Fairchild [CC BY-SA 3.0 (http://creativecommons.org/licenses/by-sa/3.0) or GFDL (http://www.gnu.org/copyleft/fdl.html)], via Wikimedia Commons

3.3 © Mark Fairchild [CC BY-SA 3.0 (http://creativecommons.org/licenses/by-sa/3.0) or GFDL (http://www.gnu.org/copyleft/fdl.html)], via Wikimedia Commons3.4 © BIO254:ORs. (2006, November 14). OpenWetWare from http://openwetware.org/index.php?title=BIO254:ORs&oldid=86883.

3.5 By The original uploader was 蔡善清 at Chinese Wikipedia [GFDL (http://www.gnu.org/copyleft/fdl.html) or CC-BY-SA-3.0 (http://creativecommons.org/licenses/by-sa/3.0/)], via Wikimedia Commons

3.6 © Hagerty Ryan, U.S. Fish and Wildlife Service [Public domain], via Wikimedia Commons

3.7 © BruceBlaus. When using this image in external sources it can be cited as: Blausen.com staff. "Blausen gallery 2014". Wikiversity Journal of Medicine. DOI:10.15347/wjm/2014.010. ISSN 20018762. (Own work) [CC BY 3.0 (http://creativecommons.org/licenses/by/3.0)], via Wikimedia Commons

3.8 © I. Ydomusch [GFDL (http://www.gnu.org/copyleft/fdl.html), CC-BY-SA-3.0 (http://creativecommons.org/licenses/by-sa/3.0/) or CC BY 2.5 (http://creativecommons.org/licenses/by/2.5)], via Wikimedia Commons

4.1 © Andreas1 (Adapted from Image:Boite skinner.jpg) [GFDL (http://www.gnu.org/copyleft/fdl.html) or CC-BY-SA-3.0 (http://creativecommons.org/licenses/by-sa/3.0/)], via Wikimedia Commons

4.2 © Pixabay

4.3 © Wolfgang Wander (Own work / http://www.pbase.com/image/83910026) [GFDL (http://www.gnu.org/copyleft/fdl.html) or CC-BY-SA-3.0 (http://creativecommons.org/licenses/by-sa/3.0/)], via Wikimedia Commons

4.3b Sonograms kindly supplied by Professor Douglas A. Nelson, Director, Borror Laboratory of Bioacoustics, The Ohio State University.

4.4 © Ken Thomas (KenThomas.us (personal website of photographer)) [Public domain], via Wikimedia Commons.

4.5 © Brian W. Schaller / License: CC BY-NC-SA 3.0 — or — FAL 1.34.6 With kind permission of Professor Tetsuro Matsuzawa, Kyoto University.

4.7 © Andres via https://www.flickr.com/photos/andreskrey/14203589736/

4.8 With kind permission of Arno Louise Meintjes.

4.9 With kind permission of the baby's mother.

4.10 © Ashby Merson-Davies. Children photographed with the kind permission of their parents.

4.11 With kind permission of Lynda Clifford, North Wiltshire U3A.
4.12 © Ashby Merson-Davies.

6.1 © Ron Knight from Seaford, East Sussex, United Kingdom (Blackcap Uploaded by snowmanradio) [CC BY 2.0 (http://creativecommons.org/licenses/by/2.0)], via Wikimedia Commons
6.2 © Sandstein (Own work) [CC BY 3.0 (http://creativecommons.org/licenses/by/3.0)], via Wikimedia Commons
6.3 © Lmbuga (Luis Miguel Bugallo Sánchez) (Own work) [GFDL (http://www.gnu.org/copyleft/fdl.html) or CC-BY-SA-3.0 (http://creativecommons.org/licenses/by-sa/3.0/)], via Wikimedia Commons
6.4 © Oregon Department of Forestry (Homestead coho salmon) [CC BY 2.0 (http://creativecommons.org/licenses/by/2.0)], via Wikimedia Commons.
6.5 Reproduced with the kind permission of the photographer Robert Joyon.
6.6 © Ashby Merson-Davies
6.7 Reproduced by kind permission of British Bird Lovers (http://www.britishbirdlovers.co.uk/)
6.8 Photo reproduced by kind permission of the photographer Paul J Willoughby.
6.9 Photo by James F. Parnell. (http://www.fcps.edu/islandcreekes/ecology/bluegill.htm)
6.10 © (Photo: Paul Hebert) [CC BY 2.5 (http://creativecommons.org/licenses/by/2.5)], via Wikimedia Commons
6.11 ©Fir0002 (Own work) [GFDL 1.2 (http://www.gnu.org/licenses/old-licenses/fdl-1.2.html)], via Wikimedia Commons.
6.12 © Tango22 (Own work) [GFDL (http://www.gnu.org/copyleft/fdl.html) or CC BY-SA 3.0 (http://creativecommons.org/licenses/by-sa/3.0)], via Wikimedia Commons